Making Sense of Omega-3s: The Good Fats

Discover how 5 calories a day can save your life™

Gretchen Vannice, MS

Registered Dietitian Nutritionist

Disclaimer:

This publication contains the opinions and ideas of the author. The information contained in this book is intended to provide helpful and informative material on the subject addressed. It is not intended to serve as a replacement for professional medical advice. The author specifically disclaims all responsibility for any liability, loss, or risk, personal or otherwise, that is incurred through the use and applications of any of the contents of this book.

The author has not received any monies or sponsorship from companies or organizations for the writing of this book.

Better Health Books
PO Box 3085
Santa Cruz, CA
95063
United States of America

For special discounts for bulk purchases of this book, contact: rd@omega3rd.com

ISBN-13: 978-1519766755
ISBN-10: 1519766750

Jill Kelly, PhD, editor
Daniel Chamberlin, layout

NOTE:

What you are about to read is documented by credible research from around the world.

For simplicity, the research is not included here but it is available either in the medical literature or from the author.

Why I Wrote This Book

I have been working with fat and nutrition research for more than 14 years. The science of nutrition is complex. We are flooded with mixed messages. Finding reliable information is difficult. As an educator, I know the confusion and how this confusion affects what we eat each day.

This book simplifies the topic of fat for you. There are fats we *need to eat*. There are fats we *want to eat*. We can have them both – really, we can - but we need more of the Good Fats. Omega-3s are the Good Fats.

In this book, you'll learn about the Good Fats. You'll learn what they are, why they are vital for your life, and how to get them in your diet without too much fuss (or cost).

My goal is for you and your family to have the lifelong benefits that the Good Fats provide.

Sincerely,

Gretchen Vannice, MS, RDN

TABLE OF CONTENTS

Quick Reference Charts

9 THINGS TO KNOW

ABOUT GOOD FAT

1. Nearly all Americans are not getting enough (and it shows).
2. The human body requires Good Fat but cannot make it so we need to eat it.
3. You need Good Fat to age well and live longer: To have better health, better sex, and to stay biologically younger.
4. Eating Good Fat is critical for your heart, blood pressure, and circulation.
5. Eating Good Fat is critical for your brain and eyes.
6. Pregnant women need Good Fat for their babies to develop normally.
7. Children are healthier, happier, and better behaved when they get Good Fat.
8. You can get Good Fat from regular food or affordable supplements.
9. Environmentally friendly and sustainable sources are available.

Good Fat, Bad Fat, What's the Story on Fat?

Most of us get plenty of fat in our diet. We like fat. We like how it tastes, how it feels in our mouth, and we like to feel full. We need fat. We need fat for our skin, eyes, hormones and all of our vital body parts, including our heart and brain. Babies need it to grow.

Here's the story: There is fat that we *must eat* and there is fat that we *like to eat*.

The *must eat* good fats are required to live full and healthy lives. Our body can't make the Good Fats so we *must eat* them. If we don't eat them, our health suffers. The Good Fats are EPA, DHA, and ALA; they are omega-3 fats. This book will tell you what they are, where to get them, and how much you need. Then it will be easy for you to get enough of the Good Fats!

The *like to eat* Okay fats are not required because our body *can* make them. We don't have to eat them but we can. Some foods that contain Okay fat are bacon, cheese, pizza, ice cream, butter, coconut oil. Of course, we don't want to eat too many calories, and fat calories add up fast. So be choosey.

Avoid trans fats. Trans fat has been manufactured for processed foods.

Fat At a Glance

Good Fats	Why we need to eat them
EAT MORE Omega-3s:	*We need omega-3s, the Good Fats, but our bodies* **cannot make** *them.* When we don't eat enough we are more likely to have heart disease, depression, arthritis, learning problems, high blood pressure, dementia, hyperactivity, anxiety, and macular degeneration.
EPA and DHA	*Sources:* Fish, fish oil, seafood, marine oils, special vegetarian supplements
ALA	*Sources:* Walnuts, flax seeds, chia seeds, avocado
Okay Fats	
EAT SOME	*We don't need to eat Okay fats because our bodies* **can make** *them.* Some is OK, but too much makes us overweight and our nutrition can get out of balance.
Solid (saturated fat)	*Sources:* bacon fat, butter, coconut oil, lard, solid cheeses, ice cream, beef fat
Semi-solid (monounsaturated)	*Sources*: Olive oil and macadamia nuts
Bad Fat	
AVOID Trans fats	*Sources:* processed foods, called 'partially hydrogenated' on labels

*Omega-3 and Omega-6 are liquid (polyunsaturated) fats. We need omega-6, too, but we get plenty in our diet. Don't worry about omega-6. Keep it simple. Eat more of The Good Fat = Omega-3.

CHAPTER 1

WHAT ARE THE GOOD FATS?

- The Good Fats are required nutrients that our body cannot make
- We need all of the Good Fats: EPA, DHA, ALA
- We especially need more EPA and DHA

Vitamins, minerals, and omega-3 and omega-6 fats are nutrients that we need to get in food and from supplements because our body can't make them. That's why they are called *essential* nutrients. For example, we need calcium for our nerves and bones and we must eat it. The same is true for omega-3. Omega-3, particularly EPA and DHA, are the Good Fats and we need them to keep our hearts and minds healthy, to have healthy pregnancies and children, and for other important reasons discussed in this book. In fact, much like calcium is part of our bones, DHA omega-3 is part of our eyes and brain.

A critical difference, however, between calcium and omega-3 is that most people know they need calcium and they get it from food or supplements. That is not the situation with omega-3. We need omega-3s, the Good Fats, and most people are not getting them. As a result, most Americans are deficient.

Bottom line: Omega-3s are *essential* for human health. They are *critical, necessary, needed*; they are *essential* fats.

There are three main omega-3s: EPA, DHA, and ALA. They are all healthful and Good Fats but there are differences in how they work in the body.

The Good Fats EPA (eicosapentaenoic acid) and DHA (docosahexaenoic acid) are directly responsible for vital, life-sustaining activities in the body, such as breathing, blood flow, and vision. They are some of the most studied nutrients in the world. The natural sources of EPA and DHA are foods from the sea.

The Good Fat ALA (alpha-linoleic acid) is another healthful fat that is important for our diet but it works differently from EPA and DHA. The natural sources of ALA are certain seeds, some vegetables, beans, and walnuts.

These Good Fats—EPA, DHA, and ALA—are all part of group of fats called omega-3s, and we need them all. However, consuming one does not replace our need for the other two. Research shows that we all need more EPA and DHA.

This might help:

Omega-3s are The Good Fats.
We need EPA and DHA Every Day.
ALA is Also good.

A bit more about the Omega-3 Good Fats

EPA and DHA and ALA are built differently from each other (in their chemistry, ALA has a shorter chain of fatty acids than EPA and DHA). This slight difference in chemistry makes a big difference in what they do in the body. In fact, while ALA has good health benefits, research shows that EPA and DHA have the greatest function; that is, EPA and DHA are the most *biofunctional*. Consuming ALA can give us a bit more EPA because ALA can change to EPA. But this doesn't happen very efficiently; less than 10% of ALA turns into EPA inside of us.

Bottom line: ALA does not replace EPA and DHA.

The other, lesser-known types of omega-3

SDA (stearidonic acid) is like ALA and a bit more efficient. SDA doesn't exist in many foods but it has been genetically engineered into soybean oil and will soon be used in foods and sold that way.

DPA is like EPA and DHA and it is also in fish. Researchers are trying to learn if it works differently or similarly to EPA and DHA. On fish oil supplement labels, it's listed as the "other omega-3."

The need for balance: omega-3 fats and omega-6 fats

Omega-6 is another type of fat, and like omega-3 it is an essential fat, but there is a big difference. See, nutrition is a bit of a balancing act. You've likely heard that it's important to balance calcium and magnesium and add vitamin D. Similarly, we need to balance omega-3 and omega-6 fats.

Most of us get plenty omega-6 fats in the food we eat but we do not get enough omega-3s. Here's why: Most processed foods, such as crackers, cookies, and chips, are made with vegetable oils. These vegetable oils (for example, soybean, safflower, and sunflower oils) contain high amounts of omega-6 fats and little or no omega-3s. So when we add together the processed foods we eat *plus* the eggs, meat, and dairy foods we eat, most of us get very high amounts of omega-6 fats in our diet.

Before we manufactured refined and processed foods, our diets contained good amounts of both omega-3 and omega-6 fats. We got omega-3s from fish, seafood, and seeds, and we got omega-6s from meats, whole nuts, grains, and seeds. We've lost the balance that is healthy for us.

For this and other reasons, it's a good idea to:

- Limit the amount of packaged, refined, and fast foods you eat.
- If you eat meat, eat moderate amounts.
- Eat more seeds and nuts, especially walnuts.
- Eat EPA and DHA omega-3 fats most days.

Eating more EPA and DHA from fish, seafood, and fish oils can dramatically improve the overall balance and give us a healthier diet. The more of the Good Fats we eat, the better we can improve the balance and reap the health rewards.

Fast Fat Facts:

- Our ancestors ate grains, beans, nuts, and seeds as whole foods. It wasn't until we learned how to press corn, soybeans, and sunflower seeds for oil that we began to eat refined oils as dressings, cooking oils, and processed foods.
- Over the past 100 years, our consumption of omega-6 fats from vegetable oils, particularly soybean oil, has increased more than 150%! while our consumption of omega-3 fats has remained about the same.
- Eating more omega-6 fats interferes with our ability to use ALA, the Also good omega-3 fat.
- Omega-6s are also essential fats, but most Americans get plenty in their diet. Some nutrition scientists report that we get far too much.
- Omega-3 fats and omega-6 fats do not change from one into the other and they do not work the same in our bodies.

CHAPTER 2

WHAT DO THE GOOD FATS DO?

- The Good Fats are required for living
- They feed our brain, fuel our hearts, and keep our joints moving
- Like calcium in our bones, the Good Fats are in our brain, eyes, and sperm

The Good Fats EPA and DHA work everywhere in the body. They work everywhere because they are in the tissues that make up our skin, blood, eyes, muscles, and more. The Good Fats don't give us a fat belly. The Good Fats work for us. Without the Good Fats, our bodies are compromised; our heart, eyes, brain, skin, muscles, and metabolism don't work as well as they could.

The Good Fats EPA and DHA even help our wounds heal, like from a cut or bruise. Some of our body parts have more of the Good Fats than others. For example, the brain, sperm, heart, and eyes hold onto more of the Good Fat DHA because they need more DHA.

Since EPA and DHA work everywhere in our bodies, it's no surprise they do so much good. Our job is to eat them. We need to eat the Good Fats because our bodies need them to work right and our bodies can't make them. Remember, our bodies can make the fat in French fries and cheese burgers and pizza so we don't have to eat these foods. We just like to. It's okay to eat some but we also need to get the Good Fats. (Hey, I didn't decide how all this works; I'm just letting you know so you can enjoy better health.)

All of the Good Fats are nutrients and they are in food; we just need to know which foods. We can also get them in supplements, like fish oil or krill oil. In addition, they are so vital for health that pharmaceutical companies are eager to make drugs with them. Researchers are looking at these drugs for several health problems, from autism and asthma to cancer, diabetes, arthritis, and many more. Doctors already prescribe one drug for people who have very high triglycerides (a form of fat) in their blood. It's called Lovaza®, and it contains EPA and DHA.

9 Things EPA and DHA Can Do
(if you get enough)
Proven benefits

1. For your heart
   - Manage blood pressure
   - Lower triglycerides (when they need lowering)
   - Increase the good cholesterol (HDL-cholesterol)
   - Reduce your odds of a fatal heart attack
   - Improve circulation
   - Help statin drugs work better
   - Keep your heart beating

2. For your mind
   - Help the mind stay clear and focused
   - Reduce mild to moderate depression
   - Help antidepressant medications work better
   - Lower anxiety

3. As you age
   - Keep your biological age younger
   - Keep your eyes healthy and vision clear

4. In pregnancy
   - Necessary for babies to develop their eyes and brain
   - Reduce risk of allergies
   - Improve chances for full-term birth
   - Reduce post-partum depression

5. For children
   - Improve ability to learn
   - Improve reading and handwriting
   - Provide key nutrients for healthy growth
   - Reduce aggressive behavior
   - Improve social and mental behavior
6. For rheumatoid arthritis
   - Reduce joint pain and morning stiffness
   - Can reduce need for some medications
7. For our intestines
   - Help heal the intestinal and colon lining
   - Calm irritable bowel
8. First Aid
   - Help wounds heal, such as cuts and bruises
   - Reduce pain and inflammation
9. For Athletes
   - Improve recovery and reduces soreness
   - Help keep concentration, vision, and strength

9 Things EPA and DHA May Do
(if you get enough)
Still being researched

1. Reduce PTSD (post-traumatic stress disorder), help TBI (traumatic brain injury), lower suicide attempts
2. Reduce dry eye syndrome
3. Improve the odds that you can delay or avoid dementia, Alzheimer's disease, macular degeneration, some breast cancers, and colon cancer
4. Help manage symptoms of type II diabetes and Metabolic Syndrome
5. Make the kidneys and liver work better
6. Improve health of our gums
7. Reduce infertility
8. Alleviate pain
9. Help us lose weight and maintain weight loss

Here's a little more on what the Good Fats EPA and DHA can do for you and your family:

For your heart

The number one killer of women and men in the United States is heart disease. Just like using the right oil in your automobiles helps them run efficiently; using the right oil in your blood helps your heart run efficiently. The car will still run for a while with the wrong oil and so will your heart. Your heart will run stronger, harder, and longer with the right oil.

EPA and DHA help your heart work better. They help your heart beat and your blood flow. If you have high blood pressure, EPA and DHA can lower it. If you have high triglycerides, EPA and DHA will lower them. They reduce the build-up (plaque) in your blood vessels, and make your good cholesterol (HDL-cholesterol) higher. However, to get these benefits, you need to get the right amount of EPA and DHA on a regular basis.

See the *How Much Do I Take* chart (on page 25).

Bottom line: None of us know if or when we may have a heart attack, but getting just 250-500 mg of EPA and DHA a day – *that's only 5 calories* – will dramatically increase your chances of surviving a heart attack. This is one of the most studied areas of omega-3s.

Scientists first learned about the benefits of fish and fish oil nearly 50 years ago. They noticed that Eskimos ate a very high fat diet but didn't get much heart disease while people in other countries, such as the United States and Denmark, who ate a very high fat diet had high rates of heart disease. So scientists being scientists investigated what was going on and discovered that the main difference was the type of fat. Eating a diet high in fat from sea foods (e.g., fish, seals) was good for the heart but eating a diet high in fat from dairy and animal meats was not. Now we know that some of this fat is okay but getting enough of the Good Fats EPA and DHA is a must.

For your mind

The brain is about 60% fat. Having a "fat head" is a good thing when it's the Good Fat. Just like calcium is part of your bones, DHA is part of the brain and your eyes. People who have more DHA in their body (and consequently in their heads), especially from a lifetime of eating fish and/or taking fish oil, have better memory, better cognition, and better brain health as they age.

You may have seen the headlines reporting that fish oil supplements don't slow cognitive decline. What's true, is that after a lifetime of not getting the Good Fats that you need, taking a supplement for a year or so after cognitive decline has started isn't going to perform miracles. Giving vitamin A pills to men who have smoked 2 packs of cigarettes a day for 20 years isn't going to perform miracles and stop cancer either. Getting more of the Good Fats at any age is smart and there are sure benefits, but prevention is best. People who eat more of the Good Fats over their lifetime have sharper minds as they age.

Another reason to get the Good Fats is to help your mood. Having good amounts of EPA and DHA in your system will improve your mood, lower anxiety, and can reduce post-traumatic stress disorder. Getting enough EPA and DHA also helps people who are depressed. It won't cure depression, nor does it take the place of a good doctor (or medicine that you need), but psychologists recognize that people who take antidepressant medication should get plenty of EPA and DHA.

Many people who are depressed don't have much of the Good Fats in their bodies; that may be because when we're depressed, we don't eat well, or because our brain needs more. We don't know for sure, but we do know that getting the Good Fats will help your brain and your nutrition. A winning combination.

Fast Fat Fact: People in other countries who eat more fish have less depression.

For your eyes: dry or degenerating

Our eyes need the Good Fat DHA just as our bones need calcium. Infants use DHA to develop their eyes while still in the womb and our eyes continue to need DHA for life. Getting more DHA in your diet reduces your risk of getting macular degeneration. For adults, getting enough of the Good Fats EPA and DHA can relieve dry eyes.

Reduce inflammation

What is inflammation? Inflammation happens when a part of body is tight, stuck, or constricted. Our tissues are always working, when we are awake or asleep: our heart beats, our blood flows, we stay warm or cool, and we breathe. These processes work because they are balanced.

The Good Fats EPA and DHA reduce the tightening and constriction that happens when we get hurt, overuse our muscles, have arthritis, asthma, irritable bowel, and more. We can also have inflammation in our blood. You may have heard that what many chronic diseases, such as diabetes, heart disease, gum disease, and obesity, have in common is *inflammation*. This internal inflammation affects our entire body and makes us sicker. We get more of this internal inflammation when we don't get enough EPA and DHA. This is one of the main reasons why we need to eat or supplement with the Good Fats. Indeed, the Good Fats are vital nutrients; we need them to keep our tissues (and our body parts) working in balance.

In addition, since EPA and DHA reduce inflammation, they are good for athletes, for first aid, and for people with rheumatoid arthritis and intestinal troubles. Having less inflammation can help several health conditions, even more than listed here. However, for EPA and DHA to work, you need to get enough and get it regularly. See the *How Much Do I Take* chart (on page 25).

Fast Fat Facts:

- Adults who added EPA and DHA supplements to their exercise program lost more weight than their counterparts who only exercised.
- DHA is part of male sperm and low amounts have been connected to infertility.
- When men have more EPA and DHA, they are stronger as they age.
- EPA and DHA can reduce our risk for cancer.
- About 84,000 deaths a year in the US could be prevented if people got the minimum amount (250 mg/day) of the Good Fats EPA and DHA each day.

CHAPTER 3

HOW MUCH DO I NEED?

- Everyone needs *at least* 250 mg of EPA and DHA each day
- Higher amounts are needed for specific health benefits
- Getting them regularly is best

The Good Fats EPA and DHA and ALA are required for living.

Knowing how much of the Good Fats you need is determined by what you already eat, how healthy you are, your family history, and other factors.

Here is a simple way to determine how much to take:

The minimum amount you need to prevent deficiency:

<u>**EPA and DHA**</u>: From age 2 to 102, you need *at least* 250 mg Every Day. *More is better.*

> You can get this much from eating certain fish twice a week and/or taking supplements, such as fish oil. Keep reading to learn how to get what you need without much fuss (or cost).

<u>**ALA**</u>: From age 2 to 102, getting at least 1,500 mg/day is Also good. More is better.

The problem:
In the US, most adults get about 100 mg EPA and DHA per day and children get less than 40 mg/day.

You can find the amount of EPA and DHA in fish in the *Good Fats in Foods* **chart on page 90.**

How Much Do I Take?

Target amounts of EPA and DHA*

Adults

For general health	At least 500 mg/day
If you have heart disease	1,000 mg/day
To lower triglycerides	2,000 –4,000 mg/day
To normalize blood pressure	2,000 mg/day
If you have mood swings	1,000 –2,000 mg/day
Depression	2,000 – 4,000 mg/day
Anxiety	2,000 mg/day
Rheumatoid arthritis	3,000 – 6,000 mg/day
Athletes	2,000 – 3,000 mg/day
Pregnancy	300 – 900 mg DHA/day
Teens	500 – 1,500 mg/day
Children:	At least 500 mg/day

*Based on current research. Your doctor or dietitian may recommend more.

How Do I Know My Good Fat Status?

The *simplest way to improve* your Good Fat status is to eat more fish or take supplements regularly. The more of the Good Fats EPA and DHA you get, the faster your status (and your health) will improve.

Guidelines to improve your Good Fat status:

- If you weigh 160 pounds or less, take about 1,000 mg EPA and DHA a day for 6 months, or 2,000 mg a day for 3 months and you will get to a basic healthy level.
- If you weigh 200 pounds or more, then you'll want to get about 1,500 mg EPA and DHA for 6 months or 3,000 mg for 3 months.

To continue to get the benefits, you'll need to continue getting EPA and DHA from food or supplements. You can maintain with 250-500 mg EPA and DHA per day. If you want more for specific health reasons, see the *How Much Do I Take* chart (on page 25). Just like vitamins and minerals, we need Good Fats on a regular basis.

Give it time.

The levels in the body don't increase overnight. Not even over a month. It takes 3- 4 months of getting EPA and DHA *regularly* for these Good Fats to get to where they work and level off. On the flipside, if you stop eating fish or taking supplements, your levels will drop.

Consume Good Fats regularly.

Whichever way you choose the get the Good Fats EPA and DHA – from food and/or supplements - do it regularly. (The EPA and DHA content of foods and supplements are in the next chapter.)

You can also learn your status with a test.

You can learn your actual omega-3 status with a test. The test measures how much omega-3 is in your blood. Most Americans have about 4%, but 8% or higher is the most protective for good health. You can do the test at home or your doctor's office. Information on at-home tests can be found in the Resource section (on page 84).

Frequently Asked Questions

My doctor has me on an aspirin a day. Can I still take fish oil?

Probably. Research shows that healthy people who take fish oil (250-500 mg/day) and an aspirin a day don't have serious problems. Getting 250 mg EPA and DHA is how much you get when you eat high quality fish twice a week, and that is recommended for everyone.

I take several prescription medications. Can I take fish oil too?

You can take fish oil. The question is how much can you take. When you eat fatty fish twice a week, you get about 250 mg EPA and DHA a day, so if you don't eat fish, taking this amount in fish oil is a good substitute. Whether you can take more fish oil depends on your health and the medications you are taking. It's always best to talk with your doctor or dietitian.

With some medicines, such as statins, getting the Good Fats is helpful and your doctor will probably recommend it. It makes sense, since statins lower cholesterol and fish oil lowers triglycerides and raises good cholesterol. It's a nice combination.

The same is true with antidepressant medications. People on antidepressants usually have low amounts of the Good Fats in their bodies. This makes sense, too, because if you are depressed, you may not be eating well. Getting more of the Good Fats EPA and DHA improves your nutrition and seems to help antidepressants work better. Another nice combination.

If you are on blood thinners, however, your doctor may advise you to limit the amount of EPA and DHA that you get over and above what you'd get from eating fish (about 250 mg/day). Then again, because of new research findings, your doctor may not advise that you limit EPA and DHA; just be sure to talk with him or her.

In general, because EPA, DHA, and ALA are the Good Fats that we need them in our diet, getting them is good for you. More can be better, but how much more depends on many things, including the foods you eat, your health, and your age.

Do I have to take fish oil every day?

It is best if you do. Just like vitamin C, our bodies need EPA and DHA every day. We need these fats regularly, from food or supplements or some of both. Aim to get some EPA and DHA Every Day and The Also Good Fat ALA most days and you'll be okay. But if you miss a day, don't worry about it. Note, however, if you are taking fish oil for a particular health condition – for your mental health, blood pressure, or arthritic pain – it's important to take the recommended amount every day. **Please don't expect results without taking the amount you need.**

Fast Fat Fact: 500 mg EPA and DHA is only 5 calories and it's all good-for-you fat!

CHAPTER 4

THE GOOD FATS AND SPECIFIC GROUPS

- Pregnant women especially need DHA
- Children and teens need more EPA and DHA
- Vegetarians and vegans need to get the Good Fats

Pregnant Women

Women who are pregnant and breastfeeding need at least 300 mg DHA a day before, during, and after pregnancy.

In the womb and during the first 2 years of life, infants need the Good Fats, especially DHA. Babies use DHA to develop a healthy brain, healthy eyes, a good immune system, and a healthy central nervous system. When the infant is in the womb mom is the only source for DHA. The infant is completely dependent on mom for the DHA and the infant will deplete mom's levels if supply is low. Mom needs to get enough DHA.

In the last trimester of pregnancy infants have a "growth spurt". This is when they need the most DHA. It is crucial that the mom gets enough DHA for herself *and* for her infant. During the growth spurt is when the infant's brain gets bigger and DHA becomes a part of the brain and the eyes. In fact, infants who are born pre-term are often fed DHA to replace what they would have received if they had been in the womb full-term.

Some nutrition scientists believe 600 – 900 mg DHA per day may be optimal. No matter what, mom needs to get at least 300 mg DHA per day.

Because the need for American women to get enough DHA omega-3 is so great, both the US Food and Drug Administration and Environmental Protection Agency recommend that women who are pregnant and/or breastfeeding eat 8-12 ounces of fish and seafood (that's 2-3 servings) every week. They recommend eating fish that is low in mercury, such as Pollock and salmon, and avoid shark, swordfish, king mackerel, and tilefish. Only one can of regular Albacore tuna is recommended per week. See the Resources section (on page 84) for information on choosing fish.

For pregnant women who won't eat fish or who only eat fish that is very low in omega-3, such as tilapia, taking a DHA supplement is a good option.

If you are pregnant or planning to be pregnant, talk with your doctor about getting DHA omega-3.

Fast Fat Fact: The baby's need for DHA is more important than mom's. If mom doesn't get what she needs, the baby will deplete her and mom is more likely to get post-partum depression. Mom needs the Good Fats to replenish herself, both mentally and physically.

Pregnant women and the Good Fat

How much do they need: At least 300 mg DHA per day

Is more better? Yes. 600 - 900 mg DHA is better

On average, how much DHA are they getting?
About 75 mg or less each day

What is the greatest concern? That all pregnant women get enough DHA for proper development of their babies and for themselves

There is special concern for pregnant women who follow vegetarian and vegan diets to get the DHA they need. Pregnant women on vegan diets have some of the lowest DHA levels *in the world.*

Finally, some women believe that eating more of the Good Fat ALA is sufficient. This is false. Pregnant women need DHA. Even if women eat large amounts of ALA, from flax or chia seeds, for example, they will not have enough DHA for their infant and themselves.

Children and Teens

All of us need to get the necessary vitamins, minerals, and essential fats to be healthy, but it's especially important that children do. From preschool to junior high, children's bodies double or triple in size. The brain continues to develop into the teen years. To grow into healthy teens, children need the right nutrition and this includes the Good Fats.

Fish has several nutrients that kids need, and it's a simple way for them to get EPA and DHA. Eggs fortified with omega-3s are a good option too.

There is so much concern that kids get the Good Fats they need that the Food and Drug Administration and Environmental Protection Agency now recommend all young children be fed fish 2-3 times a week.

In many countries, kids grow up eating fish; it's a regular food, similar to the way Americans eat chicken. Fish is accessible, familiar, and less expensive than other sources of protein. Toddlers snack on bite-size pieces; teens eat it in tacos and sandwich wraps.

Children and the Good Fats

How much do they need? At least 250 mg EPA and DHA a day

Is more better? Yes. 500 – 1,000 mg a day is better

On average, how much EPA and DHA are they getting? About 40 mg or less each day

What is the greatest concern? Poor nutrition, compromised growth, not doing well in school, increasing risk of chronic diseases in adulthood

Teens and the Good Fats

How much do they need? At least 500 mg EPA + DHA a day

Is more better? Yes. 1,000 – 1,500 mg a day is better

On average, how much EPA and DHA are they getting? About 60 mg or less each day

What is the greatest concern? Depression, early onset heart disease, and aggressive behavior

Fast Fat Fact: Kids with attention deficits and behavior problems and kids who are overweight typically have lower amounts of EPA and DHA in their bodies.

Here are some tips to help your kids learn to like fish:

- Serve a small portion of fish on the side of the plate with a familiar food, such as macaroni and cheese, and don't expect them to eat it.
- Kids usually need to see a new food 6 or more times before they will try it and like it. By the way, this is a good tip for introducing any new food.
- Start with a mild tasting fish such as Pollock or cod.
- Kids watch what others eat, especially dad and older siblings, and they follow their example.
- Be creative! Add fish to familiar foods, such as tacos, burritos, or put anchovies on pizza. Experiment! Try out different recipes and ways of making it delicious.
- Canned tuna and salmon are inexpensive and make good meat replacements in many dishes.
- If you can, make fish a regular food without fuss.
- Learning to enjoy fish is a gift that will last a lifetime.

Fast Fat Fact: Studies show that our young men and women who enlist in the US military don't have much of the Good Fats EPA and DHA in their bodies. As a result, there is grave concern over their physical and mental health while they are actively serving and when they return home. These low amounts reconfirm that most teens are not getting enough EPA and DHA.

For more sound advice on feeding children, I recommend the book 'They Are What You Feed Them', by Dr. Alex Richardson.

Vegetarians and Vegans

Everybody needs to get some EPA and DHA. Vegetarians and vegans have a unique predicament because they often eat large amounts of soy and/or soy-based foods and the fat in soy limits the effectiveness of omega-3.

Consider taking an EPA and DHA supplement or be consistent with these 3 steps:

- Eat generous amounts of the ALA from walnuts, flax seeds, chia seeds, and other foods. Chapter 6 has more on ways to get ALA.
- Take a vegetarian DHA supplement or eat foods with DHA added. [see below]
- Use olive, canola, or coconut oil in the kitchen and limit soybean, corn, and sunflower oil. If you want to avoid genetically modified oils, buy certified organic.

There is a vegetarian DHA made from algae. It is added to vegetarian and vegan snacks, milks, juices, other foods and supplements. A vegetarian form of EPA from algae is being produced and will be available soon.

Getting enough DHA is especially important for pregnant women because babies require it to develop normally while in the womb. From food or supplements, all pregnant women need at least 300 mg DHA per day.

Some simple menu suggestions:

- An easy way to get more flax and chia seeds each day is to add them to smoothies or baked goods, such as muffins or banana bread.
- Find some foods fortified with vegetarian DHA that you like and add them to your regular diet. There are many types of DHA-fortified foods available, such as juices, meal bars, and even chocolate.
- If you eat eggs, consider buying omega-3-enriched eggs.
- Toss walnuts on salads and add to baked goods. They are also a great snack and easy to transport.

Lastly, consider becoming a pescatarian and eat selected fish on occasion. See the Resource section (on page 84) about fish selection and sustainability.

Fast Fat Fact: Vegetarians and vegans have less EPA and DHA in their body than meat-eaters; one study reported 30-50% lower levels.

CHAPTER 5

HOW TO GET THE GOOD FATS
EPA AND DHA

- In food, EPA and DHA are naturally found in fish and seafoods
- EPA and DHA are added to some foods so we have more ways to get them
- Supplements, like fish oil, are an easy and reliable way to get the Good Fats

The Good Fats EPA and DHA are found in foods from the ocean, in fish and seafood. It's similar to vitamin C: Vitamin C naturally exists in citrus fruits, and so we eat oranges or drink juice to get vitamin C in our diet. We can also take vitamin C supplements or buy foods that have vitamin C added. The same is true with EPA and DHA.

You can eat food that has EPA and DHA in it naturally (e.g. fish). You can buy supplements (e.g. fish oil) or you can buy food that has EPA and DHA added to it (e.g. snack bars).

From Food

Most fish provides many good nutrients, including lean protein and trace minerals, as well as the Good Fats EPA and DHA. However, the Good Fats don't exist in all fish. There is more of the Good Fats in *fatty* fish, such as salmon, sardines, tuna, and trout. On the other hand, fish that is low in fat doesn't have much EPA and DHA in it, such as tilapia. In terms of nutrition, tilapia is more like chicken. See the amount of EPA and DHA in fish in the *Good Fats in Foods* **chart on page 90.**

Fast Fat Fact: Fish that live in very cold waters have the most EPA and DHA.

Best Fish and Seafood Sources of EPA & DHA

Wild salmon

Anchovies

Mussels

Rainbow trout

Sardines

Worst Fish and Seafood Sources of EPA & DHA

Tilapia

Catfish

Orange roughy

Scallops

Shrimp

The easiest and most affordable way to get the Good Fats is to eat fish on a regular basis. Whether that means canned salmon on salad, sushi, tuna casserole, or a snack of sardines on crackers, having fatty fish for lunch or dinner at least twice a week is best. Taking fish oil supplements works great, too, but if you eat fish, you also get protein and vitamins and minerals. Plus, it will satisfy your appetite and fill you up!

No need to go fishing, unless you want to. There are many easy ways to get fish.

Cooking fish at home

Cook fish at a high temperature for a short time, like in the broiler or on the grill.

Ways to buy fish:

Fresh vs. frozen

Fresh fish is great but it isn't available all year. The best time to buy fresh fish is when it is in season. Buying frozen fish is also a great choice, especially fish from Alaska. When fish is frozen immediately after it is caught, you get similar nutrition as buying it fresh. The nutrition is frozen into the fish. Fresh or frozen, it's best to know where the fish is coming from. You can rely on fish from Alaska. We Americans are fortunate to have great fish in Alaska.

Canned fish

There are many types of canned fish available. For example, sardines, with or without salt and sauces added, tuna, and salmon. Whether in a can or a pouch, it's a good idea to keep tuna in the kitchen cupboard and in the refrigerator so it's ready to eat. Tuna sandwiches are a favorite among many and tuna can be a great choice after school or for a late night snack. Canned salmon is another good choice for making last minute party dips and tossing into a salad.

You may have noticed that different brands of canned fish have different taste qualities. That is because there are differences in the fish and how it is handled before it is canned. Let's take tuna as an example. Canned tuna can be made from fresh tuna or from previously cooked tuna. Whether it goes into the can fresh or already cooked, it is cooked in the can. Tuna that is canned while still fresh costs more because handling fresh fish costs more (refrigeration, transport costs, etc.). Cooking tuna immediately after it is caught (before canning) makes it easier to handle and lowers the cost. This difference can impact the taste. Tuna that is cooked twice (before and after canning) will have water or oil added to the can to provide moisture during the second cooking process. Canned tuna made with fresh fish can be cooked entirely in its own EPA and DHA-rich oil. There are also differences in the amount of Good Fats. Canned tuna that has been cooked twice has less EPA and DHA than fresh canned tuna. The amount of EPA and DHA can range between 600 and 3,000 mg per 3-ounce serving. Reading the label will help guide you.

Canned salmon is usually made with fresh salmon but it can also be made with cooked salmon.

Fish in pouches

Fish packed in pouches is another great way to go. The pouches don't need to be refrigerated until after they are opened so they are convenient for traveling and taking for lunch. The pouches are especially good for kids, seniors, and for eating away from home because you don't need to use a can opener or handle anything sharp (no tools required!). The pouches are BPA-free and environmentally friendly, too. You can buy different sizes, from individual snack size to heat-and-eat family sizes of just fish or already made into soups, curries, and stews.

Note: All fish – fresh, frozen, canned, or in pouches – must be kept in the refrigerator after the package is opened.

Fast food vs. from the grocery store: Fish fillets and fish sticks

The fish used to make fillets and fish sticks is usually white fish. White fish contains some but not a lot of the Good Fats (about 100 mg EPA and DHA per serving). Buying fast food fish may be better than no fish at all, and it can be another way to help kids (and adults) become familiar with fish. Remember that the breading and deep-frying at fast food restaurants plus the sauces and dips add more fat calories (not from Good Fats), and these fat calories add-up quickly.

There are lots of choices in the grocery store freezer. You can buy fish to cook or heat-and-eat in many shapes and sizes, such as sticks, fillets, and bite-size. There are traditional breading, lightly breaded, and gluten-free choices. You can also find more varieties of fish, such as white fish, cod, Pollock, and salmon. With so many choices you'll need to read the label and find a brand you and your family enjoy.

Fast Fish Fact: A serving of frozen fish sticks usually have about 100 mg of EPA and DHA but 3 ounces of canned pink salmon can have 10 times that much.

Choosing fish to eat at home or restaurants

For help on buying fish, see the Resources section (on page 84) for tools and smart-phone apps.

Fish and the environment

The media has created fear about eating fish. Some of the information is fact-based, but much is fear-based. Fish is a valuable food source and has been for centuries. Fish caught in large open seas, such as albacore tuna in the Pacific Ocean, salmon from Alaska, and farmed rainbow trout provide great nutrition. There are some fish that we should or eat less often, such as shark, swordfish, marlin, and sturgeon. These four fish, and other predator fish, have long lives and therefore long-time exposure to potential pollutants. Avoiding these fish is especially important for pregnant women.

Based on extensive research and risk assessments, nutrition scientists agree that the benefits to our health (from eating fish) are far greater than theoretical risks. Even more important: we are paying a very high price – with our health and pocket book - from being deficient. We need the Good Fats and our body cannot make them.

Several national and international groups are working to protect the oceans and the fish and seafood that live in them. See the Resource section (on page 84) to get information about the ongoing efforts to protect our fish and oceans.

The Seafood Nutrition Partnership is a national non-profit organization focused on improving the health of the public by eating more seafood. They work with healthcare providers, national health agencies, the seafood industry, and local communities. www.seafoodnutrition.org

Bottom Line: Even if you have not been a regular fish eater, it's worth the effort to find ways to enjoy it or take supplements.

Meal ideas

Some ideas on eating fish twice a week:

	Lunch	Dinner	EPA and DHA (approximate)
Week 1	Tuna sandwich (Albacore)	Grilled salmon	1,300 mg
Week 2	Sardines on crackers	Tuna casserole (light)	1,100 mg
Week 3	Canned salmon sandwich	Anchovies on pizza	2,000 mg
Week 4	Pollock fish sticks	Fresh trout	1,150 mg

If you ate these foods, you would get, on average, about 200 mg EPA and DHA per day. You would get more EPA and DHA if you ate wild-caught tuna and salmon, fresh or canned.

More ideas:

- Salad with crab + avocado
- Fish taco or burrito made with canned or fresh fish; also a great way to use left-overs
- Appetizer plate with bite-sized fish served with cheese and crackers
- Soup made with salmon, tuna, or cod
- Caesar salad with anchovies
- Sautéed Chilean sea bass with wine and capers
- Grilled halibut dinner
- Pan-fried trout dinner
- Vegetable stir-fry with mixed fish and garlic
- Left-over fish added to salads or stirred into dips

From Fortified Foods

Foods that have the Good Fats added to them are called "fortified foods". These are foods that don't naturally contain the Good Fats but manufacturers have added them. Eating these foods is another way to get more of the Good Fats in your diet.

Foods can be fortified with EPA and DHA, or ALA, or vegetarian DHA. The only way to know which of the Good Fats are in the food is to read the label.

Omega-3 eggs

Eggs naturally contain some DHA, about 25 mg in the yolk. Eggs are also a good source of complete protein and vitamins. In addition, there are several types of fortified eggs on the market. Some are fortified with ALA and others with EPA and DHA; they type of fat in the egg depends on what the chickens are fed. The only way to know which Good Fat is in the egg is to read the label.

In general, if you eat fish a couple of times a week, you don't need to buy fortified eggs, but if you don't eat fish, then eggs that provide more EPA and DHA may be worth the higher price. Eggs fortified with EPA and DHA can be a great choice for seniors, pregnant or breast-feeding moms, and young children. ALA is easier to get in the diet, so you probably don't need to pay a higher price to get eggs fortified with ALA.

Pasta Sauce

There is a new line of pasta sauces that have EPA and DHA added. This is a simple and familiar way for the family to get more of the Good Fats.

Beverages

DHA is added to smoothies, soy milks, nut milks, and juices. You need to read the label but it is usually vegetarian DHA. There is a new flavored water with EPA and DHA added. Since the Good Fats are fat-based nutrients (like vitamin D), it's best to drink these waters with a food or snack to get the most benefit.

Snack foods

There are many snack foods on the market, such as tortilla chips and granola bars made with flax and chia seeds; these snacks contain ALA.

There are also snack foods made with EPA and DHA from fish oil. How much of the Good Fats that are in these foods varies. For example, there is a snack bar that has 300 mg EPA and DHA and a chocolate that has 300 mg EPA and DHA (in only 50 calories).

EPA and DHA are available in other foods, such as yogurt, butter substitutes, milk, olive oil, and even pizza crusts. Since food makers are also learning how important it is for Americans to get more of EPA and DHA from fish and seafood, they are experimenting with ways to add it to foods without any fish taste. More and more of these foods are coming to the market.

Finally, some foods are fortified with vegetarian DHA. There are a variety of snack bars on the market, including a line of vegan chocolate bars. If the DHA source is vegetarian, it should state that on the label.

Grass fed beef

Beef cattle raised on grass have more omega-3 in the meat, but not very much. The overall amount is still quite low; you may prefer to eat grass-fed beef, it doesn't provide much EPA and DHA.

Bottom Line: The label will tell you which of The Good Fats (and how much) are in these foods.

From Supplements

Dietary supplements from reputable companies are an easy and reliable way to get more of the Good Fats EPA and DHA into your diet. Like buying fish, there are many choices available: different sizes of capsules to swallow or chew, gummies, flavored oils (e.g., lemon cod liver oil), flavored smoothie/pudding type, and supplement meal bars.

Most fish oil supplements in the US and Canada are made from anchovies and sardines. These are smart to use because they are great natural sources of the Good Fats. In addition, the fish are small, grow quickly, are sustainable and not endangered. Plus, there is no waste: all of the fish is used because the non-oil parts go into pet foods and animal feed (animals need good nutrition, too!). You can also find supplements made from salmon, Pollock, squid (calamari), and krill.

Fish oil comes in regular or concentrated forms

Regular fish oil has about 300 mg EPA and DHA in each 1000 mg of oil. This is about how much EPA and DHA is in fatty fish, naturally.

Fish oil can also be concentrated to get more EPA and DHA in each serving. Concentrated fish oil can contain between 400 and 800 mg EPA and DHA per 1000 mg of oil (this would be 40% or 80% EPA and DHA).

Concentrated products can provide twice as much (or more) EPA and DHA than regular fish oil. They are often a better value because you get more EPA and DHA per capsule or teaspoon. Another benefit: when you get more in each serving, you can take less of it.

The only way to know how much EPA and DHA is in a fish oil (or other EPA and DHA) supplement is to read the label for the amount of EPA and DHA per serving.

Cod liver oil

Cod liver oil is a traditional remedy that doctors and families have used for centuries. Doctors gave cod liver oil to patients with rheumatoid arthritis in the 1700's. Children in northern European countries are given cod liver oil, especially in the cold winter months, because the Good Fats and vitamins A and D boost the immune system.

Liquid cod liver oil is an affordable way to get more EPA and DHA without swallowing pills. The oil is much fresher than it was decades ago, and it comes with or without natural flavors added. There are many ways to get it into your diet. You can eat lemon or orange flavored cod liver oil from a spoon, or mix it into juice, add to smoothies, or stir into pudding and yogurt. After the bottle is opened, keep it in the refrigerator.

The difference between fish oil and cod liver oil

Fish oil comes from the body of the fish and cod liver

oil comes from the liver of the cod fish. Cod liver oil also has vitamins A and D. The amount of vitamin A and D in the cod liver oil can vary by brand. Reading the label will tell you.

Krill oil

Krill are a tiny shrimp. Like fish oil, krill oil contains EPA and DHA and some of it is in a slightly different form; this different form is called a "phospholipid' form. We don't know if this difference makes any real difference in how our body uses EPA and DHA. We get the Good Fats EPA and DHA from both krill oil and fish oil and we absorb both of them quite well. What gives krill it's pink color is the natural coloring in shrimp. Some people find they don't burp when they take krill oil but this may be because krill oil capsules usually have less EPA and DHA in each capsule. Take whichever product you prefer. If you are concerned about fishing for krill, look for companies that are certified for sustainability. You can find information on the label or the company's website.

Supplement meal bar

There is a meal bar available online that tastes like an oatmeal cookie. It has 2,000 mg EPA and DHA plus vitamin D, fiber, and other good nutrition.

Storing fish oil: Capsules and liquid forms

You do not have to keep fish oil capsules in the refrigerator or freezer. You can, but you don't have to. Fish oil supplements contain natural preservatives, usually vitamin E. If keeping it in the refrigerator means that you forget to take it, then don't store it there. Instead, leave it on the kitchen counter or your desk at work. *Liquid* fish oil, however, such as cod liver oil, must be kept in the refrigerator and should be consumed within 1-2 months. Fish oil (and krill oil) should not be exposed to high heat.

Cooking with liquid fish oil

Not a good idea. Do not cook with fish oil. However, using fresh cod liver oil in a salad dressing or dip is tasty; just be sure to eat it right away.

Quality Matters

Quality manufacturing requires skill, technical knowledge, and advanced engineering. Fish oils are perishable. From the catch to the bottle, quality manufacturers take steps to keep the oil fresh and pure. Oils that are processed at high temperatures and high speeds cost less but don't have the same overall quality. They may be stripped of other nutrients, go rancid faster, and need more preservatives.

Consider this: Both whole grain flour and white flour are flour. They are both processed. One retains additional components found in its natural state (whole grain) and the other meets minimum standards (white). Fish oil products are similar. All quality fish oil products are refined, but they can be refined to meet minimum standards or meet higher standards and retain more qualities from the original source.

Independent or 3rd-party testing

Omega-3 supplements *can* be independently tested to verify they are pure and fresh and free of contaminants and that they contain the amounts of EPA and DHA stated on the label. Omega-3 companies have to pay to have this testing done and several companies do. Look for the verification or certification logo on the label. Having this testing done is voluntary; it is not required.

Here are four programs that do independent testing and report the results:

- International Fish Oil Standards™ Program
- ConsumerLab.com; access to ConsumerLab.com requires a nominal annual membership fee, about $35.00/year or so.
- NSF International
- The U.S. Pharmacopeial Convention (USP)

Each of these companies has a website that publishes the test results. See the Resources (on page 84) section.

How to Buy Fish Oil (or other EPA and DHA supplements)

Before you shop, decide how much EPA and DHA you want to get. Chapter 3 has more information. The very minimum is 250 mg per day, but it's best to aim for *at least 500 mg EPA + DHA* per day. You can also see the How Much Do I Take chart on page 25.

Read the label for:

- The serving size (it's usually 2 capsules)
- The amount of EPA and DHA *per serving*
    Note: the amount of EPA and DHA is *different* from the amount of fish oil
- Check the expiration date

You may want to consider:

- The size of the capsules
- Liquids need to be kept in the refrigerator
- Vegetarian source, if that's important to you
- Verification of independent quality testing

For example, see the label here:

- The serving size is 2-capsules
- There is 500 mg EPA and DHA per serving. Note: there is 500 mg EPA and DHA in 1200 mg of fish oil.

Next, let's calculate the price:

The bottle costs $20.00 and has 120 capsules.

There are 60 servings in the bottle.

$20.00 divided by 60 = 33 cents *per serving*.

Each 2-capsule serving of 500 mg EPA and DHA costs 33 cents per day.

Supplement Label

Fish Oil Capsules 1200 mg		
Supplement Facts		
Serving Size:	2 Softgel capsules	
Servings Per Container:		60
Amount per Serving		
Calories	24	
Calories from fat	20	
		% Daily Value
Total Fat	2.4 g	3%
Polyunsaturated fat	0.8 g	
Cholesterol	45 mg	15%
Vitamin E	3 IU	10%
Fish Oil		
EPA (mg)	300	
DHA (mg)	200	

Frequently Asked Questions

What if I have allergies to seafood?

First, work with your doctor to identify your allergy as specifically as possible. Some people are allergic to shellfish but not finfish, and vice versa. Allergens exist in the protein portion of food (e.g., meat), and better quality fish oil is purified and typically contains non-detectable levels of protein.

In reality, there is not much research, but individuals who are allergic to fish can often take purified fish oil and/or cod liver oil. Check with your doctor before experimenting. Your doctor may be able to test and confirm your allergy.

I hate eating fish but know I need the EPA and DHA.

You are a good candidate to take fish oil (or another EPA and DHA supplement) on a regular basis. Shop for foods that have EPA and DHA added, too.

Where do I buy fish oil (or other EPA and DHA) supplements?

Good question. You can buy supplements everywhere! At natural food stores, pharmacies, grocery stores, box membership stores, and online. The choices can be overwhelming. Here is what I suggest:

1. Aim for good.
    a. Buy from reputable companies at reputable businesses. Fish oil is a natural ingredient from food, so you want it to be handled right.
    b. Don't buy products from unknown sources or mysterious websites.
    c. Don't buy products from television infomercials and doctor-only "pharmaceutical grade" websites; the products are okay, but the prices are very high and you can't believe everything they say. Pay for the fish oil you need, not for celebrities and advertising.
2. Buy what you can afford.
    a. Getting some of the Good Fats is better than getting none.

b. Choose a product with a certification of quality or purity.

c. If supplements are beyond your budget, canned salmon, sardines, and tuna are a great choice and affordable. Your body will thank you.

What do I do if a capsule smells bad?

If a capsule smells bad, the oil may have become rancid. Fresh fish oil capsules will smell like fish, but they don't smell bad. You wouldn't eat bad fish; don't take bad fish oil. Check the expiration date on the bottle. Return the product to the store or toss it.

If fish oil capsules become 'cloudy' in the freezer, are they are bad?

No. Saturated fats, such as shortening and coconut oil, are solid when chilled. If your fish oil capsule is purified but becomes cloudy in the freezer, it means there is some saturated fat in the fish oil. Fish have saturated fat inside them, just like humans, so it will be in the capsule unless it's removed. If you buy supplements with more EPA and DHA, there will be less saturated fat in the capsule.

What if I burp fish oil pills?

A few people who take fish oil supplements get "fishy" burps or *repeat*. If this happens to you, try these ideas:

- Take the supplement with food, preferably the largest meal of the day.
- Do not take fish oil on an empty stomach
- Take the supplement at bedtime.
- Try enteric-coated supplements.
- Switch to flavored liquid fish oil.
- Try a different form or brand.

Of course, if you have digestive problems, consult your doctor or dietitian. In my experience, people don't usually burp higher-quality supplements.

Are fish oil and omega-3 the same thing?

Sort of. Omega-3 (EPA and DHA) is in fish oil. We take fish oil to get omega-3.

I have trouble swallowing big capsules. What can I do?

Look for companies that make small or mini capsules or consider taking a flavored liquid. FYI, if you take smaller capsules, you will need to take more of them unless you buy a product with more EPA and DHA in it. If you take a liquid, you will need to store it in the refrigerator and use within 1-2 months. You might also consider eating more fish. Tuna and salmon in cans or pouches are easy to eat year-round.

Should I take more EPA or more DHA?

We get both EPA and DHA in fish and seafood and we need both. EPA and DHA work together. However, for specific reasons, your doctor or dietitian may recommend more of one than the other. Athletes and people who have arthritis, for example, may want more EPA than DHA. On the other hand, more DHA than EPA may be what you need for your eyes and brain. Keep it simple. Taking a supplement with both EPA and DHA is a great solution for everyone.

I've been buying gummy candies with omega-3 for my family. Is this OK?

Gummy candy vitamins are sweet and easy, but they usually have a tiny amount of nutrients. Look at how much EPA and DHA is in each serving and then calculate if you and your family are getting what you need. If you regularly eat fish, then you won't need as much EPA and DHA from a supplement. However, people who need to get a specific amount of omega-3, such as pregnant women, probably won't get all they need from gummy candy vitamins.

I like to buy organic. Can I get organic fish oil?

No. Organic fish and fish oil doesn't exist. There are international standards related to the environment and sustainability. For example, the Marine Stewardship Council (msc.org) is a non-profit organization that has standards for sustainability. Looking for the MSC ecolabel™ on foods will help support global sustainability. See the Resources section (on page 84) for more information.

I want to avoid genetically modified supplements

Fish oil supplements on the market today are made from actual fish (or krill, salmon, Pollock, etc.) and are not genetically modified. However, genetically modified forms of omega-3 are being developed and will come to the market, but are not here yet

Bottom Line: We absorb omega-3s quite well from both fish and fish oil supplements. What's important is that we get omega-3s in our diets regularly.

CHAPTER 6

HOW TO GET THE GOOD FAT ALA

- The Good Fat ALA is naturally found in plant foods
- ALA is a healthy fat but cannot replace EPA and DHA
- Foods with ALA are great on salads, in smoothies, and for snacks

Walnuts, flax seed, chia seed, and some other plant foods contain the Good Fat ALA. Like EPA and DHA, we need ALA and our body does not make it. You can eat food that has ALA in it naturally (e.g., walnuts). You can buy supplements (e.g., flax seed oil) or you can buy food that has ALA added to it (e.g., snack bars).

Eating more ALA is better for you than eating more solid fats. It gives us good daily nutrition and it is good for our heart. Some research shows that ALA can reduce our risk for cancer, keep our immune system stronger, and help us maintain healthy weight. This makes sense, since ALA is in plant foods and plant foods also contain a natural mix of vitamins, minerals, fiber, some vegetable protein, and special nutrients called phytonutrients.

After you have your plan to get enough EPA and DHA in your diet, add foods with ALA. We are advised to eat less meat (or smaller portions) and eat more nuts and seeds, anyway, so eat nuts and seeds that have ALA. See how much ALA there is in seeds and nuts in the ***Good Fats in Foods* chart on page 91.**

Fast Fat Fact: EPA, DHA, and ALA are all Good Fats and we need to eat all of them. Consuming one does not replace our need for the other two.

From Food

Best Nut and Seed Sources of ALA

Walnuts

Flax seeds

Chia seeds

Hemp seeds

Butternuts

Walnuts

Walnuts are an excellent source of the ALA. In fact, walnuts are the only nut with a good amount of the Good Fat ALA. A quarter-cup of chopped walnuts has about 2,500 mg (2.5 grams) of ALA.

Walnuts are a great snack. They are easy to send in lunches, toss into salads, or take on the road. Consider giving walnuts to kids after sports practice, either alone or mixed with dried fruit. The protein they contain, along with the Good Fat, other vitamins, minerals, and phytonutrients, will be nourishing and filling. Try them toasted; spread them on a cookie sheet and cook at 350 degrees for about 10 minutes.

Keeping them cool is best: walnuts in the shell can be stored at room temperature but shelled walnuts should be kept in the refrigerator or freezer.

Flax seeds

Flax seeds are small, light brown oval seeds with a slightly nutty taste. Flax seeds are an excellent source of ALA and a good source of protein (about 20%) and both soluble and insoluble fiber. Most flax seed is grown in Canada and parts of the Midwestern USA. One tablespoon of ground flax seed has about 1,500 mg ALA.

Whole and ground organic and non-organic flax seeds are easy to find in stores. You can find whole flax seeds in packages or bulk bins. If you buy flax seeds that are already ground, be sure they are in a sealed container and keep it sealed after opening. If you want to buy whole flax seeds and grind them at home, a small blender works well. A coffee grinder that you only use for grinding seeds also works well. Ground flax seeds should be stored in the refrigerator or freezer.

Geek detail: Flax seeds are about 42% fat (by weight); about 57% of this fat is ALA. Flax is also a good source of lignans (phytoestrogens), other phytonutrients, and antioxidants. Like most seeds and nuts, they are gluten-free.

Cooking with flax seeds

Ground flax seeds can added to breads, muffins, cold and cooked cereals, and smoothies. They can be sprinkled on salads or stirred into yogurt or applesauce. Try ground flax seeds instead of flour to coat chicken before baking (it's gluten free).

Fast Fat Fact: Whole flax seeds must be chewed thoroughly or ground, otherwise they will pass through the body whole.

Chia seeds

Chia is the edible seed of the desert plant *Salvia hispanica*. These small round seeds have a slightly nutty flavor and smell. Like flax seed, chia seeds are a good source of ALA; they also contain about 15% protein and fiber (both soluble and insoluble). One tablespoon of chia seed contains about 2,100 mg ALA.

Organic and non-organic chia seeds are used in cereals, bars, snack chips, breads, puddings, and several types of drinks. They can also be added to smoothies. They do not need to be ground to get the most benefit.

Geek detail: Chia seeds are about 30% fat (by weight); about 55% of this fat is ALA. They also contain minerals, such as calcium and magnesium, and are gluten-free.

Hemp seeds

Hemp (*Cannabis sativa*) has been cultivated for thousands of years, for both the fiber and seed. Hemp contains about equal amounts of protein, carbohydrates, and fat. It is a good source of fiber (about 30%) and also contains some B-vitamins and minerals (e.g., magnesium and manganese). A quarter-cup of hemp seeds has about 1,800 mg ALA.

Organic and non-organic hemp seeds are used in snack bars, cereals, chips, breads, and drinks. They can also be added to smoothies.

Geek detail: Hemp seeds are about 30% fat, of which 15%–20% is ALA. Hemp is unique and contains two other liquid (polyunsaturated) fats: it's 2%–3% GLA (gamma linolenic acid) and 3%–5% SDA (stearidonic acid).

Avocados

An average-size avocado contains about 225 mg ALA. Half of an avocado, sliced and eaten on crackers, tossed in a salad, or made into guacamole, will add more than 100 mg of the Good Fat ALA to your diet.

Avocados are technically a fruit, but most of us think of them as a vegetable. Either way, eating avocados is a great way to get some healthy fat along with other good nutrition.

Canola oil

Canola oil has some advantages over other vegetable and cooking oils. It is low in solid (saturated) fat, has more ALA than most vegetable oils (about 11%), and is lower in omega-6 fats (corn, cottonseed, and soybean oils). If you want to avoid genetically modified canola oil, buy certified organic.

From Supplements

Flax seed oil

The oil pressed from flax seeds has a mild but slightly nutty flavor. Since the Good Fat ALA is an oil (fat), most of the ALA in flax seeds is in the oil. One tablespoon of flax seed oil has more than 7,000 mg ALA. Organic and non-organic choices are available. After the bottle of oil is open, it should be stored in the refrigerator.

Like fish oil, it is not a good idea to cook with flax seed oil. Fresh flax oil can be added to stir-fries or casseroles at the end of cooking, just before eating. It also works well in salad dressings or blended with butter and used as a spread.

WHERE DO I BEGIN?

It's best to start with the foods you already eat.

Take this simple quiz. Pick one answer for each question.

1. I eat fish
   a. Twice a week or more
   b. Maybe twice a month
   c. Never
2. When I eat fish, I eat
   a. Salmon, tuna, sardines
   b. Halibut, grouper, cod
   c. Tilapia, catfish
3. I regularly eat
   a. Flax seeds, chia seeds, and walnuts
   b. Almonds, peanuts, cashews
   c. Seeds are for birds. I don't eat any

If you mostly answered A's, you are getting what you need daily from your food. If you want more of the Good Fats for any health reasons, take a supplement.

If you mostly answered B's, either start eating more fish or take an EPA and DHA supplement, such as fish oil.

If you mostly answered C's, run to the store and get a EPA and DHA supplement and start eating walnuts, too.

Bonus points: Find out what your own status of the Good Fats is today. Do it yourself with an at-home test (see Resources section on page 84) or ask your doctor for a test.

RESOURCES

At-home omega-3 testing

These tests measure omega-3 status with a drop of blood; it's the finger-prick method:

Holman Omega-3 Test®
http://www.omega3test.com

Omega-3 Index
http://www.omegaquant.com

Fish and seafood recommendations

The Environmental Working Group has tools to calculate your own seafood list to help choose seafood that is lower in mercury, higher in the Good Fats omega-3 and sustainable.

Seafood calculator:
http://www.ewg.org/research/ewg-s-consumer-guide-seafood/seafood-calculator

Seafood guide:

http://www.ewg.org/research/ewgs-good-seafood-guide/executive-summary

The Monterey Bay Aquarium Seafood Watch® program rates fish and seafood by environmental impact.

Consumer Guides:

http://www.seafoodwatch.org/seafood-recommendations/consumer-guides

The app:

http://www.seafoodwatch.org/seafood-recommendations/our-app

Environmental Defense Fund Seafood Selector
http://seafood.edf.org/

The US Environmental Protection Agency Fish Consumption Advisory:
water.epa.gov/scitech/swguidance/fishshellfish/fishadvisor ies/

Fish4Health

Find state-by-state fish consumption advice.

http://fn.cfs.purdue.edu/fish4health/

Independent product quality testing

ConsumerLab.com

Independent tests and reviews of vitamin, mineral, and

herbal supplements

http://www.consumerlab.com/

International Fish Oil Standards™ Program (IFOS™)

Testing Services: IFOS and QC Program

http://www.nutrasource.ca/ifos/

NSF® International

http://info.nsf.org/Certified/Dietary/

USP: US Pharmacopeial® Convention

http://www.usp.org/dietary-supplements/overview

Sustainability and environmental resources

The Environmental Defense Fund works to preserve oceans and is a good resource for learning about fish and the environment.

http://www.edf.org/

The State of Alaska Fish Monitoring Program routinely monitors salmon, halibut, Pacific cod, Pollock, and other marine and freshwater fish from coastal waters throughout the state for trace minerals and possible pollutants. Detailed reports of the testing results are available at:

https://dec.alaska.gov/eh/vet/fish.htm

The Marine Stewardship Council (MSC) is a global nonprofit organization working to protect and sustain the world's seafood supply. Fish and seafood that meets their standards will have a MSC ecolabel™ on the package. You can look for the label in grocery stores and restaurants. There is a link at www.msc.org to locate local MSC-certified foods.

Energy & Environmental Research Center is a leader in environmental research and technologies and provides environmental and nutritional resources.

http://www.undeerc.org/fish/

Where to find nutrition research

Office of Dietary Supplements: National Institutes of Health

http://ods.od.nih.gov/

PubMed: US National Library of Medicine: Medline

http://www.ncbi.nlm.nih.gov/pubmed

Registry and results database of private and public clinical research studies

https://clinicaltrials.gov/

Good Fats in Foods

Amount of EPA and DHA in Fish

Fish (per 3 ounce serving)	EPA (mg)	DHA (mg)	Total
Chinook salmon	858	618	1475
Bluefin tuna	310	970	1280
Pink salmon (canned)	450	630	1080
Sockeye salmon	450	595	1045
Rainbow trout	284	697	981
Sardines (canned)	400	433	833
Albacore tuna (canned)	198	535	733
Sea bass	175	473	648
Halibut	77	318	395
Light tuna (canned)	40	190	230
Grouper	30	180	210
Haddock	65	138	203
Atlantic cod	0	130	130
Tilapia, farmed	5	59	64
Catfish, farmed	7	30	37

Source: USDA

Amount of ALA in Seeds and Nuts

Food	How much	ALA (mg)
Flax seed, oil	1 tbsp	7,260
Flax seed, ground	1 tbsp	1,550
Chia seed	1 tbsp	2,100
Walnuts, chopped	¼ cup	2,660
Butternut	¼ cup	2,600
Hemp seed	¼ cup	1,800
Canola oil	1 tbsp	1,280
Canola oil, high oleic	1 tbsp	308
Pecan, chopped	¼ cup	270
Pistachio	¼ cup	80
Pumpkin seed, roasted	¼ cup	33
Cashew, chopped	¼ cup	22
Peanut, Spanish	¼ cup	4
Peanut, Valencia	¼ cup	4
Almond, slivered	¼ cup	3

Source: USDA
Seeds and nuts are raw unless stated otherwise.

INDEX

ABOUT THE AUTHOR

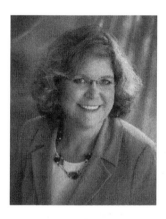

Gretchen Vannice, MS, RDN, is an independent nutrition consultant, educator, author, and speaker based in Northern California. She is a recognized expert in omega-3 nutrition.

She was the lead author of the Position Paper for the Academy of Nutrition and Dietetics on Dietary Fatty Acids for Healthy Adults and is a member of the Scientific and Nutrition Advisory Council for the Seafood Nutrition Partnership.

She is a resource for health professionals, researchers, and the omega-3 food and supplement industry.

Visit her website: www.gretchenvannice.com

Photograph: Mark Comell

Other recent publications by Gretchen Vannice

Boost your Omega-3s in *Diabetes Living Magazine*. 2015.

Dietary Fatty Acids for Healthy Adults in the *Journal of the Academy of Nutrition and Dietetics*. 2014.

A Ridiculously Easy New 9-Switch Plan to Build Muscle, Not Belly Fat in *Prevention Magazine*. 2014.

Omega-3 Handbook, A Ready Reference Guide for Health Professionals. 2011.

Medical Nutrition Therapy for Psychiatric Conditions in *Krause's Food and the Nutrition Care Process* 13th ed. 2011.

Omega-3s from Fish and the Risk of Metabolic Syndrome in the *Journal of the Academy of Nutrition and Dietetics*. 2010.

www.gretchenvannice.com

Made in the USA
Lexington, KY
01 April 2017